YOUR KNOWLEDGE HAS VALUE

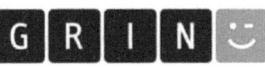

Bibliographic information published by the German National Library:

The German National Library lists this publication in the National Bibliography; detailed bibliographic data are available on the Internet at http://dnb.dnb.de .

Imprint:

Copyright © 2016 GRIN Verlag, Open Publishing GmbH
Print and binding: Books on Demand GmbH, Norderstedt Germany
ISBN: 9783656985624

This book at GRIN:

http://www.grin.com/en/e-book/333870/cast-study-critique-report-on-francis-report-2013-recommendation-15

Kamalesh Dey

Cast Study Critique Report on "Francis Report 2013 (Recommendation 15)" About Mortality Statistics

GRIN Publishing

GRIN - Your knowledge has value

Since its foundation in 1998, GRIN has specialized in publishing academic texts by students, college teachers and other academics as e-book and printed book. The website www.grin.com is an ideal platform for presenting term papers, final papers, scientific essays, dissertations and specialist books.

Visit us on the internet:

http://www.grin.com/

http://www.facebook.com/grincom

http://www.twitter.com/grin_com

University of Bedfordshire

Business School

MBA (HOSPITAL AND HEALTH SERVICES MANAGEMENT)

ORGANISING MODERN HEALTH CARE SERVICES

CAST STUDY CRITIQUE REPORT

ON

"FRANCIS REPORT (RECOMMENDATION 15)"

BY

KAMALESH CHANDRA DEY

08 May 2016

WORD COUNT: 3100

EXECUTIVE SUMMARY

The report explored the Francis report regarding Mid Staffordshire NHS Foundation. The report also examined and analysed the recommendation 15 of Francis report based on Mid Staffordshire NHS Foundation. The report mainly highlighted the mortality statistics of the Mid Staffordshire NHS Foundation and how mortality statistics influenced the entire hospital as well as NHS foundation trust through the different performance strategies. Mortality statistics was done through data collection, data analysis, assessing hospital performance, and publishing the final audit report, while the report highlighted that auditing was the best strategy to improve the total performance of the hospital.

In addition, the critique report recommended seven principles for medical auditing for instances clinical and health providers individual's duty, self-management of the medical staffs, availabilities of the auditing, essential criteria of the auditing, required resources of the medical auditing, record keeping, and evaluation of the final audit outcomes by various medical and non-medical experts. These seven principles were identified as effective and significant to provide the quality care of the patients and improve the overall performances of the medical organisations.

CONTENT

Table of Contents	Page No

INTRODUCTION

The report will explore the Francis report regarding Mid Staffordshire NHS Foundation. The report will also examine and analysis the recommendation 15 of Francis report based on Mid Staffordshire NHS Foundation. The report will particularly highlight the mortality statistics of the Mid Staffordshire NHS Foundation and how mortality statistics can influence the whole organisational structure and help to improve the hospital performance (attached is appendix 1). In addition, the critique report will recommend some of the significant strategies to improve the quality of the services of Mid Staffordshire NHS Foundation.

The Mid Staffordshire NHS Foundation Trust was a NHS foundation trust and managed two hospitals named Stafford and Cannock Chase Hospital in Staffordshire, England. However, Stafford Hospital was quite bigger (350 inpatient beds) and Cannock Chase Hospital was a bit smaller (115 inpatient beds). In 2008, the trust was awarded as a NHS foundation trust, while in 1993 it was named Mid Staffordshire General Hospitals NHS Trust and around 3,000 employees worked in the two hospitals (Healthcare Commission, 2009). Unfortunately, there was a scandal reported in Francis report. The report published that there were about 400 to 1200 deaths at the Mid Staffordshire NHS Foundation Trust due to poor quality care, lack of facilities and failures of medical treatment between 2005 and 2009. Therefore, Government had taken that case as serious issues and organised an independent investigation. Francis was appointed for this investigation and completed by 2011. After investigation, he published his full 2000 pages report in 2013 and divided into three volumes. He also provided almost 290 recommendations (Francis, 2013).

Francis outlined 290 recommendations in his full report. Recommendation 15 is about Mortality statistics. The analytical report will analyse recommendation 15 and identify as how Mortality statistics can support and influence to improve the quality of the hospital performance through regular data collection, data analysis, assessing hospital performance including medical and non-medical staffs, publishing final outcomes in various media and journals (attached in appendix 1). The Mid Staffordshire NHS Foundation Trust was in dreadful condition in term of quality performance and they failed to serve the quality of care to the patients. Publication of the Mortality statistics in the public report would play significant role to improve the hospital performance (Lindenauer et al., 2007). In addition, assessing staff performance and record the death rate in the hospital would be crucial to influence their high performance along with high quality of patients care (Marshall et al., 2000).

ANALYSIS

This section will explore the recommendation 15 of Francis report and critically analysis the effectiveness of the mortality statistics to improve the hospital performance. Mortality statistics could be done through various protocols for instances data collection, data analysis, assessing hospital performance, and finally publishing outcomes in the mass media or journals (shown in figure 1). As a policy maker, under the department of health, could imagine the following effective strategies what could be implemented in the national health industry (NHS) particularly the Mid Staffordshire NHS Foundation Trust. The following analysis would be supportive to improve the quality of the hospital performance through the addressing all the existing problems in the light of Francis recommendation 15. The key analytical descriptive criteria are described below:

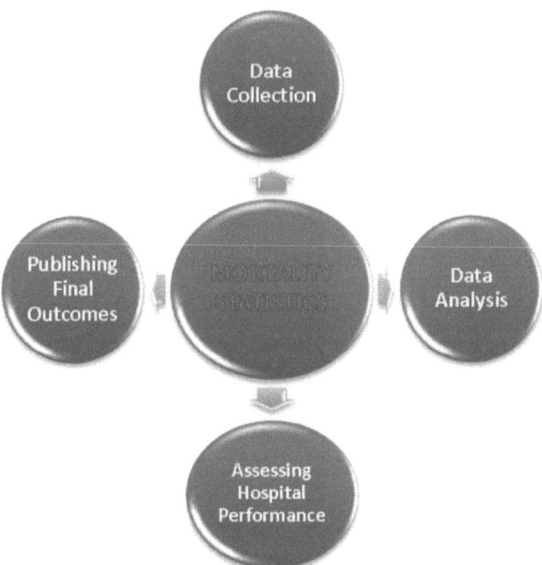

Figure 1: Mortality Statistics Protocol (Francis, 2013)

DATA COLLECTION

Data collection is very crucial to investigate or inquiry or do research on any kind of health or business industry. Lindenauer et al., (2007) stated that data collection is the best way to justify the subject areas or assessing the performance of any staff or hospital or industry. For example: Francis investigated on the Mid Staffordshire NHS Foundation Trust and finally outlined his report, while he initiated his first steps through data collection before assessing the hospital performance.

Data could be collect through numerous ways for instance survey or feedback. Survey could be done through the distribution of questionnaires or interviews like face to face, telephone, or Skype interview (shown in figure 2). Survey could be done monthly or annually.

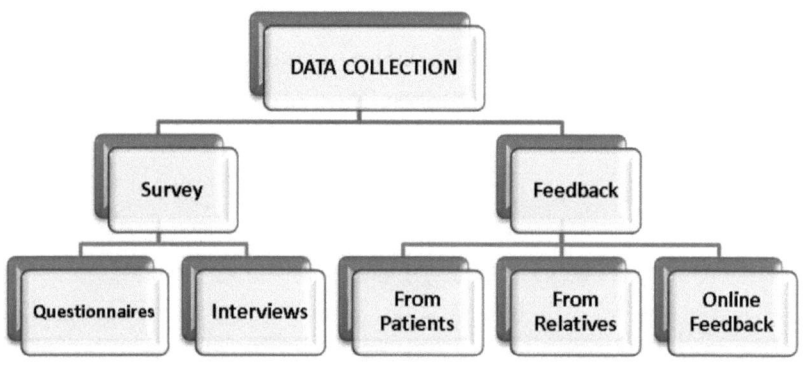

Figure 2: Data collection process (Lindenauer et al., 2007).

In addition, data could be collected through feedback from patients during discharge from the wards, relatives or hospital visitors in online survey. After getting survey result, hospital authority could know the deaths rate, drawbacks, and performance of their quality of the care. Based on their quality ratings, hospital authority would take initiative to improve their performance in term of quality of care. Therefore, mortality statistics through data collection might influence the hospital overall performance.

DATA ANALYSIS

Data analysis is very significant for the health research. After data collection, data should be analysed to get desirable outcomes or main findings (Shiloach et al., 2010). Once data collection is done, then data would be ready for analysis to get full idea about the consequences of the hospital critical issue or development of the hospital performance. Data analysis could be done through mainly three ways for instances specialist data analyst, data assessment, and data interpretation (Shiloach et al., 2010). After data collection from the hospital, data could be analysis through various agents. Suitable and meaning full data analysis makes research outcomes realistic and feasible.

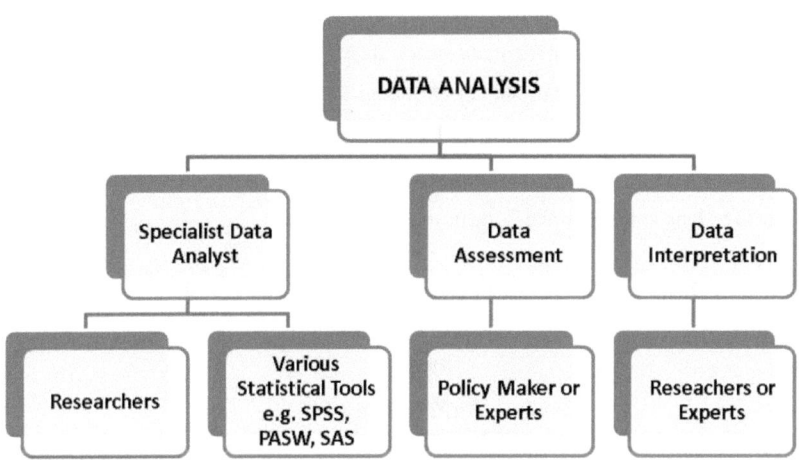

Figure 3: Data Analysis Process (Shiloach et al., 2010).

Death rate could be analysed based emergency department performance, conditions of the patients, treatment facility, and quality of care. In addition, hospital overall performance including Doctors, Nurses, HCAs, Dieticians, physiotherapist, pharmacist individuals performance might be assessed through data analysis (shown in figure 3). Researchers, data analyst, policy maker would be involved to analyse the data through numerous suitable statistical tools like SPSS, PASW or SAS (Binu, Mayya and Dhar, 2014). This analysis would provide total overview as how is hospital performing. If death rate is high then need to take initiatives against weakness or where lack of motivation or performance is involvement.

ASSESSING HOSPITAL PERFORMANCE

Assessing hospital performance is the vital part to improve the quality of the hospital. There are numerous body could be involved with this assessment to make valid outcome to avoid any types of biasness. Internal and external body could take part actively to appraise the performance in the hospital. For instances CQC (Care Quality Commission), internal hospital audit, department of health (DOH), Local Government, Local Volunteer Organisations (shown in figure 4) (Peterson et al., 2006).

CQC could inspect the hospital from top to bottom for instances quality of care, staff skills and performance, food and nutrition of the patients, hospital hygiene, infection control, fire safety measures, pest control, update record of the medical devise, staff validation documents, training up to date, patients feedback, death rate in each ward, conditions of the of the patients (Shaw and Costain, 1989). Based on all those conditions as well as mortality statistics, CQC could make their suitable score and that score would be valid until next year and if any weakness then that would be done within the provided timeframe. CQC ratings would be helpful to know about the hospital performance.

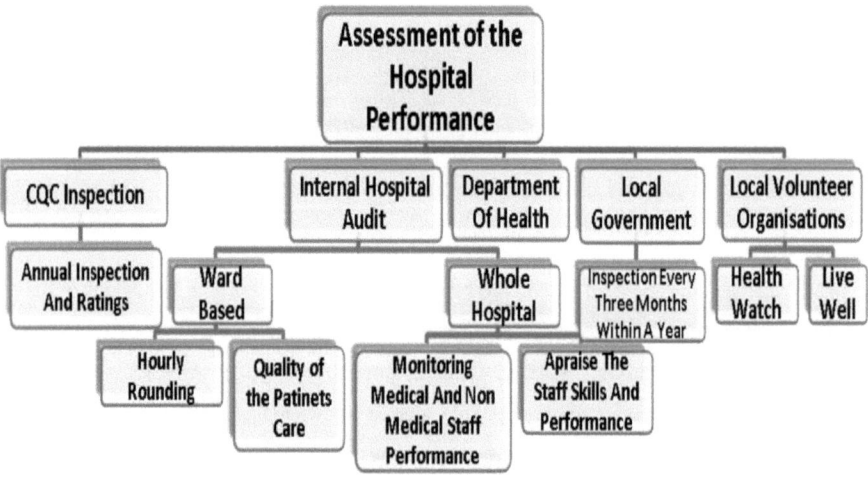

Figure 4: Hospital Performance Assessment Protocol (Peterson et al., 2006)

Internal audit is also another assessment body but it is actually under internal assessment. This is very significant for the hospital authority to know their own performance before publishing in the public place and before that they could resolve their problem without publishing. It could be ward based as well as based on whole hospital. In the ward based assessment, nurse in charge could be mentors and lead the team to assess the individual ward performance for instance hourly rounding, food and fluid chart, checking the patient weight, their treatment plan and overall the patient satisfaction score during discharging from the ward. Nurse in charge or ward manager could perform this audit on the day to day basis (Shaw and Costain, 1989).

Similarly, internal auditing based on mortality statistics and patients' safety is very crucial to assess the overall performance and quality of the organisation. Effective and frequent auditing of patient safety and management body ought to be appraised to achieve better position in the health industry. Based on case study, there was huge debate was involved in management section and significant evidence of the ignorance of their duty and responsibilities to conduct the regular auditing in the hospital and appraise the staff performance. Francis (2013) reported that Non-executive member of the hospital of Mid Staffordshire NHS foundation trust even did not visit the hospital as well as ward in person and he used to reply on third person in term of reporting and inquiry.

In addition, the management body had no especial health background apart from Sir Stephen Moss. The aim of the early auditing of the death rate and patient safety could support to identify the current problems and also helped to improve the services. It was noted that frequent auditing much effective rather than annual auditing. Hanskamp, Sebregts et al. (2013) purported that frequent audit of mortality ratio and patients safety is supportive to appraise the hospital performance for instance more death rate denotes that poor quality or care or treatment failures. These points could influence the policy to put in place on time to turn forward the hospital performance.

Likewise, all other ward could perform same ways to assess the rest of the wards in the hospital. In addition, mentors or senior in charge of the hospital could monitor the all medical and non-medical staff from Doctors, Nurse, HCAs, Pharmacist, and Physiotherapist performance. They could appraise the staff skills and performance. Hospital could organise internal training to retrain the staff to enhance staff skills before involving   any kind of accident. This is way internal audit could be done in the hospital. Shaw and Costain (1989) stated that internal audit is the best audit to improve the hospital performance as it helps to appraise the staff and whole hospital performance and there is more likely to get better performance after internal audit without any kind of penalties.

Department of health (DOH) could be involved directly with the inspection of the hospital as well as all NHS foundation trust. DOH could also monitor patient safety and put the patient first in the health services. Quality of the care would be improved if Mid Staffordshire NHS Foundation Trust follow the ideal principle and put patient first in their service then quality and performance could be developed easily (Department of Health, 2013).

Local Government could also be involved to inspect the quality and monitor the performance of the local hospital. Staffordshire local Government would initiate to visit the hospital and make formal inspection in every three months a year. Local Government audit report might be supportive to improve the performance through the addressing the findings involved with negative consequences. In addition, local volunteer organisation like Health Watch, Live Well would also inspect the local hospital to assess their performance, what could be helpful to validate the final audit and there would a chance of biasness (Lindenauer et al., 2007).

PUBLISHING FINAL OUTCOMES

Publication is the most significant part of the health research to explore the update about the subjects. Research or any kind of investigation is meaningless without publication in the public site. During the scandal of Mid Staffordshire NHS Foundation Trust, publication was the only responsible to publicise the news. For example: Francis investigated the case but without publication no one knew about the scandal.

Therefore, publication is most significant and crucial for the research. Auditing data publication is essential to increase or develop of any hospital or medical institute or medical services (Millar, Freeman and Mannion, 2015). Publication of the final outcomes could be done into three ways for instances publish internationally, nationally and locally (Marshall et al., 2000). The following process (shown in figure 5) could be followed during the publication of the outcomes:

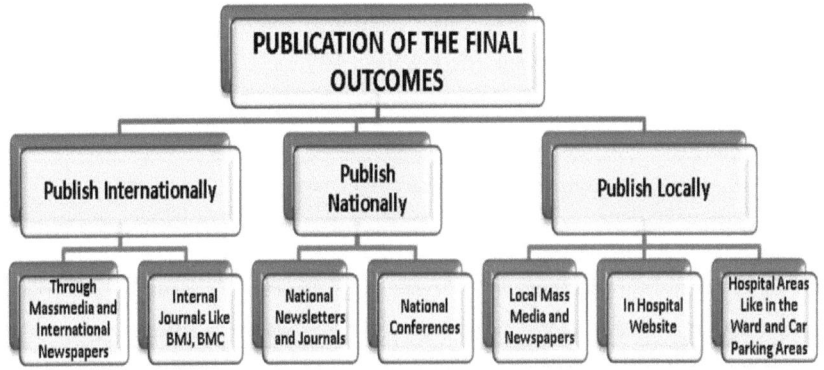

Figure 5: Publication Process of the Audit Outcomes (Marshall et al., 2000).

International publication can play vital role to improve the quality of the hospital performance. All the investigation could be published internally to get more recognition and popularity regarding the report where more people would involve directly or indirectly to develop the hospital performance through the addressing the most common drawbacks. The hospital report could be published through mass media like BBC world news and various popular newspapers like Guardian newspaper.

In addition, hospital audit report could be published various popular international journals for instances British medical Journal, BMC and various international data base like PubMed. This would be very effective to explore the audit report all the over world. Therefore, the report could bring much attention for the public as well as for the Government due to its publication (Millar, Freeman and Mannion, 2015).

Moreover, national publication is also significant to improve the hospital performance. National publication could be performed through national newsletters, journals, and presenting auditing report in the national conference where health ministry or policy maker would be present. Therefore, country policy leader or health lead could get in touch the about the real scenario of the particular hospital. Consequently, Government leader could take action against the problems of the hospital and initiate new policy in place to address the weak points in the health services in the hospital. This would be best possible importance for publishing audit report nationally (Marshall et al., 2000). For example: something was going wrong in the Mid Staffordshire NHS foundation trust and death rate was going high to higher. Afterwards, Francis investigated the case based on hospital and published as a formal report. Afterwards, it worked very well to get actively involved the health ministry to the hospital services and motivated to conduct further investigation what actually helped to find out the actual problem. Consequently, the hospital performance was getting better after addressing the existed problems in the hospital (Francis, 2013).

Furthermore, local publication is also crucial for further development of the hospital. This is actually fundamental publication of any types of health industry. Actually, publication begins from local to international, while local publication would be effective to solve the problem internally very quickly before making any kinds of historical scandal. Local publication could be done through local mass media, hospital websites, and hospital areas like car parking and various wards notice boards. Particularly, staff notice board is very effective to put the audit report, where staff could be aware about the current quality status of the hospital. This notice board report might help the staffs to motivate themselves and to push hospital performance quality forward through working hard as a team and applying their leadership skills (Millar, Freeman and Mannion, 2015).

CONCLUSIONS

The critical analytical report highlighted the recommendation 15 of Francis report regarding Mid Staffordshire NHS Foundation Trust. Mortality statistics was the noteworthy recommendation of the Francis report. Mortality statistics could be performed through various ways, what explored in the analysis report. Based on the analysis report, mortality statistics actually helped tremendously to improve the quality of hospital performance. Based on Francis report, it was noted that there were numerous internal problems going on in the trust. Therefore, they failed to control their quality in every level of the staffs for instances doctors, nurses, HCAs as well as management body in the hospital trust.

Consequently, the death rate was higher rather than any other hospitals in the United Kingdom. Lack of internal auditing, lack of staff skills influenced the death rate in the hospital. Initial mortality statistics would be supportive to resolve the problem and safe innocent life. Overall, the analysis report appraised the recommendation 15 and also added some strategic pathways along with mortality statistics to improve further developments of the quality of the hospital performance.

RECOMMENDATIONS

The following recommendations (shown in figure 6) could be followed systematically to improve the hospital performance through providing of quality care and maintaining patients safety:

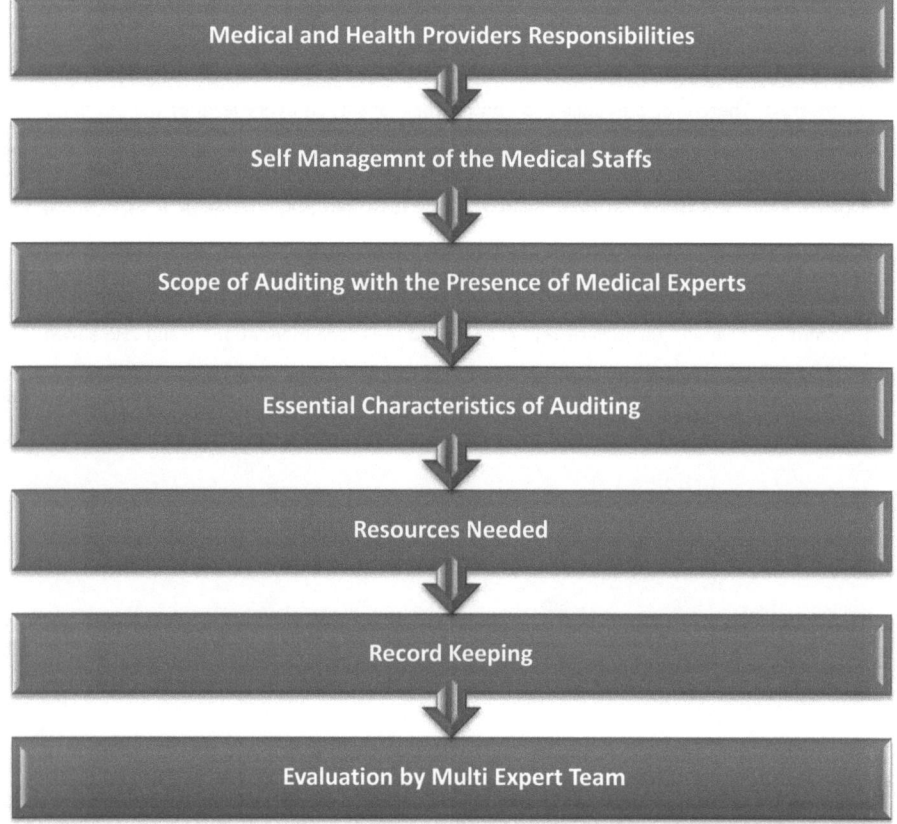

Figure 6: Recommended Seven Principles of Medical Audit for the Performance Management in the Hospital (Shaw and Costain, 1989)

Based on the seven principles of the medical audit (Shaw and Costain, 1989), hospital performance would be improved systematically. Initially, health providers and baseline medical staffs need to define clearly and more specifically disclose their individual duty in term of quality of the patients care. Secondly, clinical staffs like Doctors and Nurses should manage themselves to perform their individual duty through auditing and improve their performance through additional action if necessary. Thirdly, regular auditing program should be organised in every hospital and medical expertise must be participated in those program based on their availabilities.

Fourthly, audit should be specific, repeatable, reliable, and durable what would be supportive to change the hospital performance and their medical practise. Fifthly, medical experts and physicians need to be distributed required elements for the medical audit. Lastly, all the medical audit, process and outcomes should be recorded. Finally, audit need to be evaluated by the experts, medical team, organisational manager, and ministry of national health. The seven recommended principles would be supportive and effective to provide quality of the patients care and improve the overall hospital performance.

REFERENCES

Binu, V.S., Mayya, S.S. and Dhar, M. (2014) 'Some basic aspects of statistical methods and sample size determination in health science research', *An International Quarterly Journal of Research in Ayurveda,* 35 (2), pp.119

Department of Health (2013) *Patients First and Foremost: The Initial Government Response to the Report of the Mid Staffordshire NHS Foundation Trust Public Inquiry.* London: The Stationery Office.

Francis, R. (2013) *Report of the Mid Staffordshire NHS Foundation Trust Public Inquiry,* London: The Stationery Office.

Hanskamp-Sebregts, M., Zegers, M., Boeijen, W., Westert, G.P., van Gurp, P.J. and Wollersheim, H. (2013) 'Effects of auditing patient safety in hospital care: design of a mixed-method evaluation', *BMC Health Services Research,* 13 (1), pp.1 [online]. Available at: http://eds.a.ebscohost.com/eds/pdfviewer/pdfviewer?sid=639e2a17-3be8-4583-97b6-c3c1de7bfdae%40sessionmgr4001&vid=0&hid=4203&preview=false (Accessed: 02 May 2016).

Healthcare Commission (2009) *Investigation into mid staffordshire NHS foundation trusts.* London: Commission for Healthcare Audit and Inspection.

Lindenauer, P.K., Remus, D., Roman, S., Rothberg, M.B., Benjamin, E.M., Ma, A. and Bratzler, D.W. (2007) 'Public reporting and pay for performance in hospital quality improvement', *New England Journal of Medicine,* 356 (5), pp.486-496 [online]. Available at: http://www.nejm.org/doi/pdf/10.1056/NEJMsa064964 (Accessed: 05 May 2016).

Marshall, M.N., Shekelle, P.G., Leatherman, S. and Brook, R.H. (2000) 'The public release of performance data: what do we expect to gain? A review of the evidence', *Jama,* 283 (14), pp.1866-1874

Millar, R., Freeman, T. and Mannion, R. (2015) 'Hospital board oversight of quality and safety: a stakeholder analysis exploring the role of trust and intelligence', *BMC Health Services Research,* 15 (1), pp.1-12 [online]. Available at:

http://eds.a.ebscohost.com/eds/pdfviewer/pdfviewer?sid=0e43c290-71c4-4f1c-b3f3-4b25b405f933%40sessionmgr4001&vid=0&hid=4202&preview=false (Accessed: 01 May 2016).

Peterson, E.D., Roe, M.T., Mulgund, J., DeLong, E.R., Lytle, B.L., Brindis, R.G., Smith, S.C., Pollack, C.V., Newby, L.K. and Harrington, R.A. (2006) 'Association between hospital process performance and outcomes among patients with acute coronary syndromes', *Journal of American Medical Association,* 295 (16), pp.1912-1920.

Shaw, C.D. and Costain, D.W. (1989) 'Guidelines for medical audit: seven principles', *British Medical Journal (Clinical Research Ed.),* 299 (6697), pp.498-499 [online].Available at: http://www.bmj.com/content/bmj/299/6697/498.full.pdf (Accessed: 02 May 2016).

Shiloach, M., Frencher, S.K., Steeger, J.E., Rowell, K.S., Bartzokis, K., Tomeh, M.G., Richards, K.E., Ko, C.Y. and Hall, B.L. (2010) 'Toward robust information: data quality and inter-rater reliability in the American College of Surgeons National Surgical Quality Improvement Program', *Journal of the American College of Surgeons,* 210 (1), pp.6-16 [online]. Available at: http://ac.els-cdn.com/S1072751509014082/1-s2.0-S1072751509014082-main.pdf?_tid=913e5a6a-1302-11e6-8d85-00000aacb361&acdnat=1462481423_b05234be7cff2ca2734a9ac6454d938a (Accessed: 04 May 2016).

BIBLIOGRAPHY

Cavendish, C. (2013) 'The Cavendish review: an independent review into healthcare assistants and support workers in the NHS and social care settings', *London: Department of Health.*

Clwyd, A. and Hart, T. (2013) *A review of the NHS hospitals complaints system: putting patients back in the picture.* London: Department of Health.

CQC (2016) *Care Quality Commission appoints first National Guardian for the freedom to speak up in the NHS.* Available at: http://www.cqc.org.uk/content/cqc-appoints-first-national-guardian-freedom-speak-nhs (Accessed: 5 may 2016).

Davies, N. (2015) 'Lessons from school: what nurse leaders can learn from education.' *Nursing Management,* 22 (4), pp.34-38 [online]. Available at: http://eprints.kingston.ac.uk/32063/1/Davies-N-32063.pdf (Accessed: 04 May 2016).

Fawcett, T.N., Holloway, A. and Rhynas, S. (2015) 'If I have seen further it is by standing on the shoulders of giants: finding a voice, a positive future for nursing', *Journal of Advanced Nursing,* 71 (6), pp.1195-1197 [online]. Available at: http://0-eds.a.ebscohost.com.brum.beds.ac.uk/eds/command/detail?sid=28ca5803-6fc9-444f-a603-e19a99487732%40sessionmgr4003&vid=1&hid=4208 (Accessed: 02 May 2016) .

Forde-Johnston, C. (2014) 'Intentional rounding: a review of the literature', *Nursing Standard,* 28 (32), pp.37-42 6p [online]. Available at: http://0-eds.a.ebscohost.com.brum.beds.ac.uk/eds/pdfviewer/pdfviewer?sid=672aaedb-d667-4aed-9032-4993a3392770%40sessionmgr4005&vid=2&hid=4208 (Accessed: 03 May 2016)

GMC (2015) *Openness and honesty when things go wrong: the professional duty of candour.* Available at: http://www.gmc-uk.org/DoC_guidance_englsih.pdf_61618688.pdf (Accessed: 5 May 2016).

Halligan, A.W.F. (2014) 'Implications for medical leaders of the proposed Duty of Candour', *Clinical Risk,* 20 (1), pp.29-31 3p [online]. Available at: http://0-eds.a.ebscohost.com.brum.beds.ac.uk/eds/pdfviewer/pdfviewer?sid=e045786b-3726-4819-8734-2c2d12595642%40sessionmgr4003&vid=2&hid=4208 (Accessed: 02 May 2016).

Hutchison, J.S. (2016) 'Scandals in health-care: their impact on health policy and nursing', *Nursing Inquiry,* 23 (1), pp.32-41 10p [online]. Available at: http://0-eds.a.ebscohost.com.brum.beds.ac.uk/eds/command/detail?sid=ca3032c4-1a31-44e4-9f35-89f731a0315f%40sessionmgr4002&vid=1&hid=4208 (Accessed: 04 May 2016).

Jarman, B. (2013) 'Quality of care and patient safety in the UK: the way forward after Mid Staffordshire', *Lancet (London, England),* 382 (9892), pp.573-575 [online]. Available at: http://www.thelancet.com/pdfs/journals/lancet/PIIS0140-6736%2813%2961726-2.pdf (Accessed: 01 May 2016).

Keogh, B. (2013) *Review into the quality of care and treatment provided by 14 hospital trusts in England.* London: NHS England.

Lewis, I. and Lenehan, C. (2012) *Report of the children and young people's health outcomes forum.* London: Department of Health.

Meade, C.M., Bursell, A.L. and Ketelsen, L. (2006) 'Effects of nursing rounds: on patients' call light use, satisfaction, and safety', *AJN the American Journal of Nursing,* 106 (9), pp.58-70 [online]. Available at: https://facweb.northseattle.edu/nwhittier/NUR%20228/NURSING%20ROUNDS%20ARTICLE.pdf (Accessed: 03 May 2016).

Mitchell, M.D., Lavenberg, J.G., Trotta, R.L. and Umscheid, C.A. (2014) 'Hourly rounding to improve nursing responsiveness: a systematic review', *The Journal of Nursing Administration,* 44 (9), pp.462-472 [online].Available at: http://www.ncbi.nlm.nih.gov/pmc/articles/PMC4547690/pdf/nihms715187.pdf (Accessed; 02 May 2016).

Paul, C. (2000) 'Internal and external morality of medicine: lessons from New Zealand', *British Medical Journal,* 320 (7233), pp.499 Available [online].at: http://0-www.ncbi.nlm.nih.gov.brum.beds.ac.uk/pmc/articles/PMC1127535/pdf/499.pdf (Accessed: 02 May 2016).

Qc, R.F. (2014) 'Duty of candour', *Clinical Risk,* 20 (1), pp.1-3 3p [online]. Available at: http://0-eds.a.ebscohost.com.brum.beds.ac.uk/eds/pdfviewer/pdfviewer?sid=94f1d87c-b7d0-47cf-930a-1786631093b2%40sessionmgr4002&vid=2&hid=4208 (Accessed: 01 May 2016).

Reeves, S., Ross, F. and Harris, R. (2014) 'Fostering a 'common culture'? Responses to the Francis Inquiry demonstrate the need for an interprofessional response', *Journal of Interprofessional Care,* 28 (5), pp.387-389 3p [online]. Available at: http://0-eds.a.ebscohost.com.brum.beds.ac.uk/eds/pdfviewer/pdfviewer?sid=7ec112b6-d6ef-49ea-91ae-cb68b5dd5a9d%40sessionmgr4005&vid=2&hid=4208 (Accessed: 03 May 2016).

Roberts, D.J. (2013) 'The Francis report on the Mid-Staffordshire NHS Foundation Trust: putting patients first', *Transfusion Medicine,* 23 (2), pp.73-76 [online]. Available at: http://0-eds.a.ebscohost.com.brum.beds.ac.uk/eds/pdfviewer/pdfviewer?sid=dba90110-f02a-484c-9bed-7c15d2db0647%40sessionmgr4003&vid=2&hid=4208 (Accessed: 02 May 2016) .

Runciman, W.B. and Merry, A. (2003) 'A tragic death: a time to blame or a time to learn?', *Quality and Safety in Health Care,* 12 (5), pp.321-322 [online].Available at: http://www.ncbi.nlm.nih.gov/pmc/articles/PMC1743757/pdf/v012p00321.pdf (Accessed: 05 May 2016).

Sinclair, C.M. and Manitoba. Provincial Court (2000) *The report of the Manitoba Pediatric Cardiac Surgery Inquest: an inquiry into twelve deaths at the Winnipeg Health Sciences Centre in 1994.* Winnipeg: Provincial Court of Manitoba.

Snelling, P.C. (2013) 'Ethical and professional concerns in research utilisation: intentional rounding in the United Kingdom', *Nursing Ethics,* 20 (7), pp.784-797 [online]. Available at: http://nej.sagepub.com/content/20/7/784.full.pdf (Accessed: 02 May 2016).

Teasdale, G. (2002) 'Learning from Bristol: report of the public inquiry into children's heart surgery at Bristol Royal Infirmary 1984-1995', *British Journal of Neurosurgery,* 16 (3), pp.211-216 [online]. Available at: http://0-eds.a.ebscohost.com.brum.beds.ac.uk/eds/pdfviewer/pdfviewer?sid=5ac1212d-69a4-4b63-a5b3-81ed8bd829b1%40sessionmgr4002&vid=0&hid=4208 (Accessed: 05 May 2016).

Walshe, K. and Shortell, S.M. (2004) 'When things go wrong: how health care organizations deal with major failures', *Health Affairs (Project Hope),* 23 (3), pp.103-111 [online]. Available at: http://0-eds.a.ebscohost.com.brum.beds.ac.uk/eds/pdfviewer/pdfviewer?sid=00a72dc4-48dc-4b14-824c-46d5e73f23be%40sessionmgr4001&vid=2&hid=4208 (Accessed: 06 May 2016) .

Willis, E., Henderson, J., Couzner, L., Toffoli, L., Verrall, C., Blackman, I. and Hamilton, P. (2015) 'Rounding, work intensification and new public management', *Nursing Inquiry* [online]. Available at: https://www.researchgate.net/profile/Julie_Henderson2/publication/279177532_Rounding_work_intensification_and_new_public_management/links/55e2bc6808ae2fac471f997c.pdf (Accessed: 02 May 2016).

APPENDIX

APPENDIX 1: MIND MAP OF FRANCIS REPORT

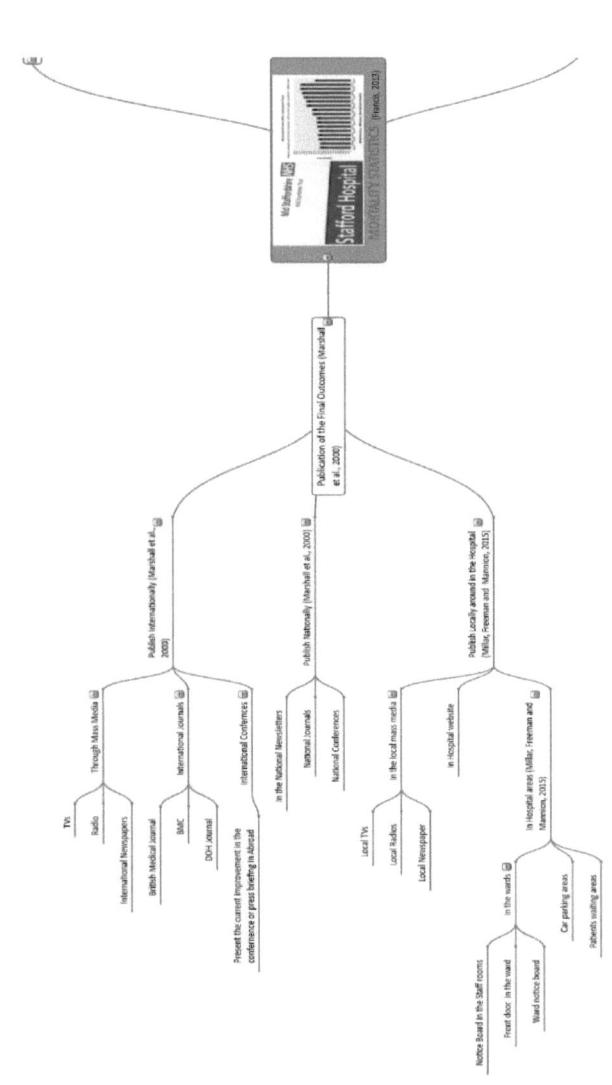

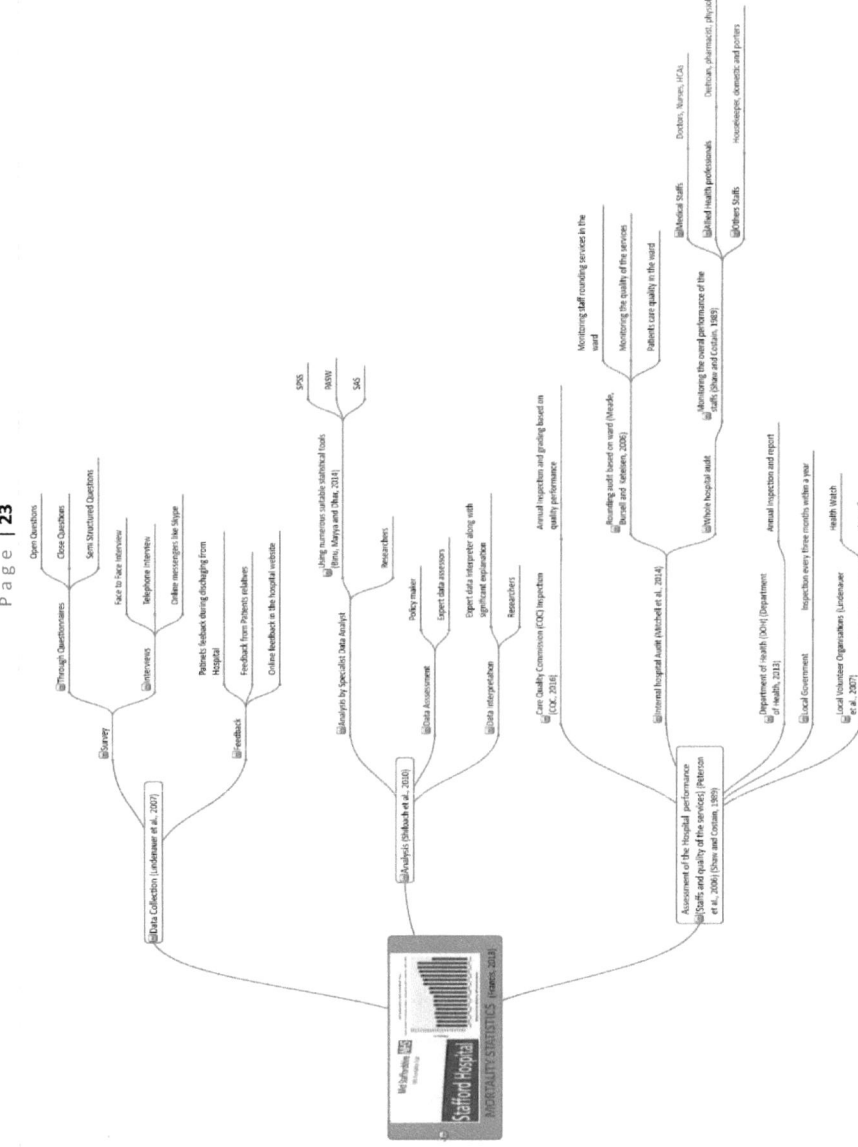

Figure 1: Mind map (in two parts) of Francis report based on the recommendation 15 (Francis, 2013)

YOUR KNOWLEDGE HAS VALUE

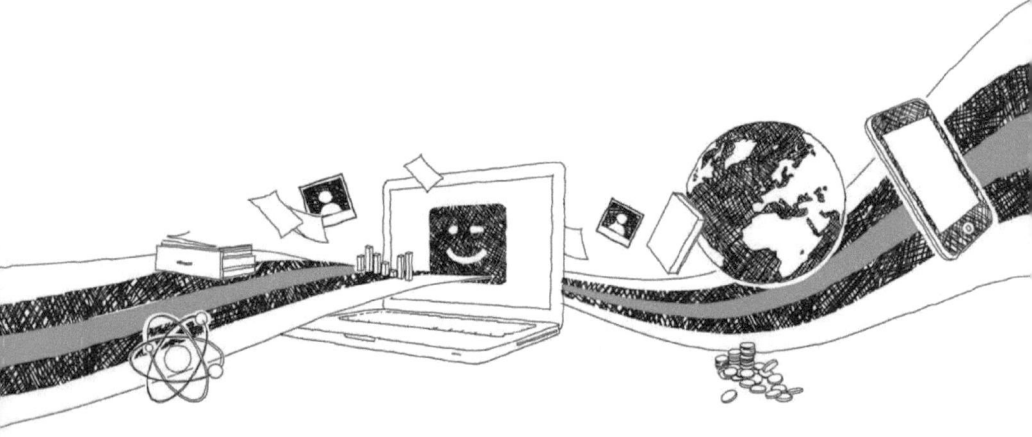

- We will publish your bachelor's and
  master's thesis, essays and papers

- Your own eBook and book -
  sold worldwide in all relevant shops

- Earn money with each sale

Upload your text at www.GRIN.com
and publish for free

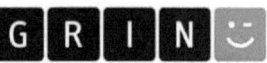